Wool-Gathering
with
The Wolf

Lina Lazaretto

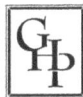

Grosvenor House
Publishing Limited

The right of Lina Lazaretto to be identified as the author of this
work has been asserted in accordance with Section 78
of the Copyright, Designs and Patents Act 1988

The book cover is copyright to Lina Lazaretto
Cover artwork by Angela Finch

This book is published by
Grosvenor House Publishing Ltd
Link House
140 The Broadway, Tolworth, Surrey, KT6 7HT.
www.grosvenorhousepublishing.co.uk

This book is a work of fiction. Any resemblance to
people or events, past or present, is purely coincidental.

A CIP record for this book
is available from the British Library

Paperback ISBN 978-1-83615-405-1
eBook ISBN 978-1-83615-406-8

For Wendy with love and gratitude.

Fortiores Una.

Contents

Preface

It's Christmas 2024 in Italy, high in the Abruzzo mountains, and I am ensconced in my ancestral village. For days it has snowed heavily, the air crisp and the sky an unholy blue. In the distance sits the Maiella Mountain, called the Mother Mountain by the ancient Oscan people, and named for Maia, the Goddess of Spring, warmth, and growth. The glittering snow blankets her like polished diamonds, the light so bright it hurts your eyes, and the need for sunglasses a necessity, not just Italian brio. At dusk and dawn the calling of the wolves bounces off the mountains and echoes through the icing sugar-coated pine forests. My days are filled with chopping wood for the open fire, then carrying it up the outside spiral staircase into the house, and checking that the feral orchard cats, who save us from summer snakes, are warm, fed, and tucked away in their straw-filled, homemade "cat apartments".

Some of my father's friends and cousins watch me as I energetically excavate a car from a huge mound of snow. Sweating and flushed, only as it is completely uncovered do I see that it is the wrong car! My mother's Fiat Panda is sitting under the adjacent icy hillock. They tease me relentlessly but usefully tell me to just uncover the number plate next time.

I am happy, fit, and healthy.

In mid-January I return home to London with a sore knee that is difficult to bend. A few weeks later, I discover a lump in my left groin. An appointment is made with my GP, who assures me that it's probably nothing and I, too, believe I have just overdone things. By mid-February I have been diagnosed with malignant tumours under my left kneecap and groin. My world changes, and the word lymphoma becomes part of my new vocabulary.

For the first chemo session, my consultant advises that I need to be hospitalised and monitored for any adverse reactions. I have never been an inpatient before; ultimately, it will be a three-and-a-half week stay. I decide in gratitude and respect to the staff who are caring for me that I will learn to say "thank you" in each of their languages.

My experience in hospital is sometime heart-wrenching, but other times gut-bustlingly funny. Occasionally, the Janus nature of humanity, fragility, and strength surfaces; a sharp reminder least you forget your predicament. I find that to surrender your adult self into the hands of complete strangers, who then cradle and care for you at you most vulnerable, is both humbling and frightening. There is camaraderie with fellow patients, so emotive and deep. Then, devastatingly, you realise you will be unlikely to see them again or know what happens to them.

As I regaled my friends and family with these tales, they cajoled me into writing them down. So here is my little book, which I hope that you will read: tales of humour, humanity, and humility on just one South East London Hospital ward.

A Note on my Chosen Nom de Plume
and Book Title

A Lazaretto is a quarantine station for travellers, which can be a building, ship, or isolated island. I read Michael Rozen's poem "Island of Strangers", and this very much fitted with my experience of my care by the staff in the ward, so the use of Lazaretto seemed fitting.

I have called the book *Wool-Gathering with The Wolf.* The idiom wool-gathering can mean daydreaming or aimless thought. In thirteenth century England, and still in modern-day Italy, the perceived connection between the devouring behaviour of the wolf and the progress of malignant cancers was so evocative that "wolf" was and is still used as a synonym for cancerous disease. As my Italian relations and friends heard of my diagnosis, each uttered the phrase "In bocca al lupo" which translates to "into the wolf's mouth". The expression compares a challenging situation to being caught between the jaws of a wild beast. The standard reply is "Crepi il lupo", meaning "May the wolf die". It seemed appropriate to have the name of the "lupo" mentioned in the title of my book. Dramatic yes, but if you can't be dramatic in times like this, then when can you be?

The Goat and The Fish

It's 6.30am, and the world has a pinkish glow from the rising sun climbing over the London streets. The curtains are still pulled around our bed bays as the night shift nurses bustle around trying to finish up before their fresh-faced colleagues arrive for the day shift by 8am.

Across the way, in the opposite corner bay to mine, Eszter, the wispy Hungarian recovering crack addict, is humming. This is not a good sign. She has learnt via Duolingo to say "I am not a morning person", and she means it. "The prickers" are about to arrive in our bay. They arrive promptly each morning to prick our fingers for blood sugar levels, stick thermometers under tongues, and thrust needles into our unsuspecting still sleepy veins. Often, they get short shrift from Eszter, who berates them like some wizened Zaza Gabor.

"Vi you vake me up? You come later – oh my life."

So, the humming is ominous, like a beehive just before a swarm.

As a distraction, I call out, "Jo reggelt" (Good morning in Hungarian), hastily learnt on Google Translate. The humming stops abruptly.

"Vatever," comes back the reply, but I can hear the intrigue in her voice.

Eszter has a lot on her mind. Elfin-like, she gives off a tough, slinky-malinky vibe but has a vulnerability that breaks your heart. Arriving here six months ago, barely alive, and just 38kg with a stomach that was about to disintegrate, she is homeless, and all her meagre possessions are pooled around her bed. She knows that she needs a complex operation to survive and to avoid eating pap for the rest of her life. Although her English is not bad, and she tries to improve it through Duolingo, the "medispeak" of the doctors confuses her. And she knows when she is discharged, she will be sent to a hostel full of "junkets", as she calls them. She is terrified. So, the "vatever" reply is good.

There is a pause, then she says, "Bed 11, vat are you?"

"Eh, what?" I reply.

"Zodat. Me, I am fish."

I understand. "Oh, zodiac signs. You are Pisces, fish. I am a Capricorn. A goat, Eszter."

There is no reply, but I hear muffled sobbing.

"Are you ok?" I ask.

"Too much. Dis my live, vat can I do, where I go, I will die!" she says.

"Eszter, perhaps try to think of just one thing at a time, otherwise it's too much. Look, be more like a goat, like me. One step, one step slowly up the mountains, instead of a fish swimming about crazy in the water."

She seems to take this to heart, and for the rest of the day all is calm.

The next morning, just before "the prickers" arrive, Eszter calls out, "Bed 11, today I will be goat!"

I agree enthusiastically. "Good, Eszter. More goat, less fish!"

When a passing nurse raises her eyebrow, with a look of "what are these crazies up to now?", Eszter catches my eye, and we dissolve into giggles.

Fishcakes and Cauliflower

"Ere, ere, you next door – you got a phone charger?" comes a voice from the next-door bay. There is a curtain between us, so I can't see the owner of the voice.

"Yes," I say. "I don't know if it will fit your phone, but we can give it a try."

A nurse goes by and is collared. "Ere, take this next door to 'er, will yer? Tar."

The nurse brings through a battered pink Nokia. Miraculously, the charger fits and it starts to power up.

"Tank you. Ere, what's yer name?"

"Lina," I say. "What's yours?"

"Dina?" she says.

"No, Lina," I reply.

"Alrite then. I'm Gladys."

I haven't met Gladys; she was wheeled in about 1am this morning, plucked from her little council flat in Catford. She explained to me later that the neighbour upstairs had a leaking pipe, and the floor in her flat was soaking wet. She had tried to put newspaper down to mop it up, but it caught around the wheels of her Zimmer frame. Taking a bad fall, she knocked herself out, leaving her with a purple "Tom and Jerry" bump and bruised forehead. Since she was admitted, they have also discovered the wolf has her – lung cancer.

With the excuse of visiting the loo, I take my crutches and hobble past her bed to get a better look.

"Hello,"I say. "I'm Lina from next door with the phone charger."

I see a frail, tiny woman, probably in her eighties, propped up in bed. She has grey-black hair down to her shoulders, as straight as a yard of pump water. Her voice, like iron railings, suits her, and her high sharp cheekbones means that she was probably "a bit of a looker" in her day. Steely grey-blue eyes take me in, suspicious, checking me, and then deciding that I'm probably alright to get to know. A slight shrug seems to say I might just be useful to her. She finally says, "Tanks for fixin' me phone, Anna."

I don't have the heart to correct her.

The food trolley lady, Patty, arrives, pushing her trolley with its noisy wheel into our bay. Eating breakfast, we are asked to choose food for today's lunch and dinner. Each week a huge, laminated menu card appears, with an array of stodgy nursery food. The "healthier options" are written in large, bold coloured font as a way of enticing us to choose wisely.

Patty goes to Gladys first, in the misguided belief that she will be a pushover.

"What would you like, dear? says Patty.

"Got any fishcakes?" says Gladys.

"No. There is…" Patty reels off a list of today's offerings.

"I'll 'ave Shepherd's pie. Have you got any cauliflower?" asks Gladys.

"No cauliflower," says Patty.

I don't realise at the time, but the request for fishcakes and cauliflower becomes a daily mantra of Gladys's. For a solid two weeks there is no sign of these delicacies, until one morning I spy fishcakes on the lunch menu.

"Gladys, they have fishcakes for lunch!" I say, not able to hold back.

"Oooh," comes the owl-like reply.

The anticipated moment comes, and Gladys says, "I'll have fishcakes."

"Yes," Patty says, "we have fishcakes."

Two women in the bay and I say "hooray", with Eszter opting for "hoorah" instead.

Gladys laughs then says hopefully "Cauliflower?"

"No cauliflower," says Patty.

However, amazingly, at the end of the week, cauliflower appears on the menu like some divine apparition. We wait expectantly in our curtained areas as Patty says, "Gladys, today we have cauliflower!"

We hold our breaths in anticipation, and there's a gameshow-length pause from Gladys. Then we hear her say, "I'll have an 'am sandwich."

Patty clicks, sucks her teeth, and with a sigh moves off. On the other side of the curtain, I silently cheer on Gladys's chutzpah and comic timing.

Jollof Rice

It's two thirty in the morning, my leg is twitchy, and I can't sleep. I have tried to get off for hours, but even my usual "go-to" of Ludovico Einaudi's complete works is not cutting the mustard, and slumber eludes me. Out of boredom, I decide to visit the loo. Peeping out into the corridor, I check who is at the nurses' station. There are some of my favourite, gregarious Nigerian nurses – Florence, Blessings, and Bola. They look up, startled; for once, it is a quiet night.

"Are you ok? Do you need help?" they ask immediately, concerned.

I nod that I'm fine. Then say, "Pele o bawo ni?" (Hello, how are you?)

My parents lived in Lagos in the sixties, working for the British High Commission. The High Commissioner enjoyed his food, and my father – a great chef – was duly employed, despite being an Italian national. It was the time of the independence and a joyous place to be. My parents, then only in their mid-twenties, had a wild time which they never forgot. I grew up listening to Nigerian Highlife music and hearing some Nigerian words that they remembered fondly and would occasionally drop into conversations. These became "family" words, that I assumed as a child only my parents, my sister, and I understood. It was only as I grew that I realised it was not a secret tongue but a real ancient, spoken language. These words retained their mysticism for me and reminded me of the joyfulness that my parents radiated when they uttered them, reminiscing on their wild times in Nigeria.

"E, you know Yoruba." The nurses laugh.

"A few words only, but you can teach me how to say thank you and a few greetings."

So, they teach me "shay" or "o shay" for thank you. But Florence is Igbo, and she says thank you is "daalu". A squabble starts as to whether Igbo, Yoruba, Hausa, or any other Nigerian dialect would be more beneficial for me to learn. I promise to learn all but think it's safer to change the subject before a mini war breaks out.

"So," I ask mischievously, "does anyone have a good recipe for jollof rice?"

"Eeh," says Bola, "you cook jollof rice?"

"Well," I reply, "my neighbour Joe cooks jollof. He says his is the best because it's his mother's recipe, but I wouldn't dare cook it. I'm Italian not Nigerian! After all," I say jokingly, "you wouldn't cook pasta, would you?" They laugh and shake their heads.

Blessings says, "Ah, so you are Italian. If I was born again, I would want to be an Italian woman – so chic."

I look at her and say slowly, "Ah, if I was born again, I would want to be an African woman."

I dance slowly, swinging my hips, and they fall about laughing. As I toddle back to my bed with my twitchy leg, I can still hear them saying, "She wants to be an African woman" and chuckling. But I fear I would never make the grade.

Gladys and Her Sisters

Gladys's family were all born and bred in Deptford. Her father and brother worked at the docks. All the families that lived in the little brick houses knew each other and everyone else's business. She went to school with Sissey and Pat. Sissey later became a bee-hived market trader in Catford, and Pat sold pints of cooked prawns outside a local drinking hole.

Gladys said of Pat, "I never liked 'er, she was a bitch." There was clearly history there, but I didn't like to ask.

Gladys's family are close, and the ancient Nokia bears testament to that, as it starts to trill at seven thirty each morning on the dot. A mind-numbing ringtone sounds out, reminiscent of "Hello Barbie, Let's Go Party". But it couldn't be, could it? The rest of the ward groans.

"Is that you?" bellows Gladys. "I can't 'ere yer, Else! Talk up, talk up. What? Nah, she dinent, did she? Fuckin hell – never – well, that's what I said. S'exactly. U coming up 'ere wid me stuff? Alrite, see yer later."

The Nokia goes off again. "Fucking hell," utters Gladys in a theatrical whisper, but she is clearly enjoying the attention. "What? Nah she can't. What she wanna another one for? She already got three kids. S'exactly!"

The calls go on for another hour, with Gladys sagely dishing out advice to her family and friends, all punctuated with her trademark "S'exactly!" and followed by "Hello Barbie, Let's Go Party" signalling the next incoming call.

Visiting hours start at 3pm, and on the dot Gladys's elder sister Else arrives. She barks at Gladys, "Ow yer doing, you alrite? I bought you some barley water."

"Nah," moans Gladys, "what yer bought me that for? Yer knows I 'ates it. I wanted Rib-eena! Tastes like bloody mouldy lemon – 'orrible!"

"Well, I fuckin bought it fer yer, and y'ell 'ave it," says Else, not swayed at all.

In one foul swoop, our elder doyen of the ward is promptly boxed and turned into a brattish, put-upon younger sibling. Curiosity gets the better of me, and I stumble out of my curtained bay heading for the loo, walking slowly on my crutches so I can get a look at Else. I think I have double vision, as I see an exact version of Gladys, a twin helping of Lizzy Dripping.

Else shoots me a look that would curdle milk and I, shockingly, realise that Gladys is the "softer" of the two.

Gladys says, "This is the lady that 'elped me wid me mobile, Else."

Else nods "ello".

I spot a young man sitting on a stool by the bed playing a casino betting game on his phone.

"That's Jack," says Gladys. "E doesn't say much. Not a blabby, are yer, Jack?" He nods without looking up, and I continue on my way.

I hear Gladys behind me, "Yeah, she's alrite. I-talian. Don't know why she's 'ere. Lezza, I fink."

The next day Jo, Gladys's younger sister. and her husband, Tel, arrive.

"Alrite, Tel," says Gladys. "Ello, Jo, dinint tink yer were coming."

Jo looks nothing like her two impish sisters. She is rotund, with a coiffured head of over-red hair and M&S frippery of best blouse and slacks.

"Whatcha bought us then?" says Gladys hopefully.

"Well, we couldn't carry much, because we've been shopping, and we can't stay long because Tel needs his tea. You know how he gets if he doesn't eat," Jo answers. "So, here's some Opal Fruits and some Bombay mix."

As soon as they leave, Gladys is on the phone to her eldest sister, Else.

"Couldn't bring me much – they got a bleedin' car! Fucking Bombay mix, I arks you! I arks'd for bloody salt 'n' vinegar crips. S'exactly – must 'ave had them in the back of 'er cupboard! Couldn't stay long because Tel needed his dinner – fucker! Nah, I dinint say nufin'. If she's 'avin an affair, it's 'er look out, she always was a cutty anyways," she goes on, her voice getting higher.

"A, whatcha mean? She never won 'alf a ton, ave yer seen it? Fifty quid! I don't believe 'er. Wot a bitch! S'exactly."

Later that evening, when the hustle and bustle of the day has passed and the ward is quiet, I pass the bottom of her bed.

"Your sister doesn't look like you or Else, does she?" I remark.

Gladys fixes me with a stony stare and barks, "She's the milkman's."

My Favourite Vampire

It hadn't been a good morning so far. A pasty-faced youth had turned up on the ward as the daily "pricker". He seemed to be suffering from the effects of the night before, was decidedly queasy looking, and green about the gills.

Shoelaces undone, he promptly knocked over the empty vials on his phlebotomist cart, scrambling to collect them before they hit the floor.

"Hello, I'm Dave, come to do your bloods," he said hoarsely "Where do you want them done?"

I raised an eyebrow. "Um, well, wherever you can get it from."

He decided on the right arm, missed the vein, went for the left and missed again.

"That's it, I can only do it twice," he said.

Thank God for that, I thought.

He moved off to the next victim but could not get blood from any of the five of us on the ward, which meant more work for the nurses later. I hoped to never see him again and, luckily, I never did.

Two student nurses decide to have a go getting some blood from me. They grab my left hand, but never over fond of needles, I am now as stiff as an ironing board, and my veins refuse to give up anything. I am left with a pulsating bruise on my hand, which will take a week to fade. Suddenly, ninja-style, a new nurse appears at my bedside. She is wearing a mask, but I can see she is probably South Asian. Her eye makeup is amazing, making her look like a masked version of the Goddess Shiva.

From her pocket she produces a small torch, then gently takes my right arm. Running the torch up and down, she locates the perfect vein, which is some feat. I have been told by many, mistakenly, that I have "good veins" as they are visible, but not one of the buggers is straight. Getting a cannula or a needle into them is always a challenge and perpetuates my general loathing of needles. I am mesmerized by this nurse and her near-magical powers; I am starting to believe she may indeed be the real Shiva. The needle is in, blood taken, and she pats my arm and says, "There," before disappearing.

"Who was that?" I ask the two student nurses who have been watching.

"Ah, that was Shevanti," they answer in a sort of awe-struck reverence.

Shevanti instantly becomes my favourite vampire; the nickname sticks, and we will meet often during my stay.

The Habit of Nunning

Eszter has had a bad few days and has asked for a visit from the local Catholic priest. He arrives, neat and polished, and pulls the curtain around her bed space, gently nudging her belongings out of the way with his toe. Usually she has no visitors, so his appearance is noted, especially by the overzealous young woman in the corner of our ward. Eszter and I had previously tried to talk to her, but it had not gone well.

Having learnt the word zodiac on Duolingo, Eszter decided it was a good starting point for a conversation, rejecting the usual British dissociated but polite weather conversations.

"Hello, I am Eszter, I am a piece," she says enthusiastically.

The young woman looks up. "Eh?"

"Hi, I'm Lina. Eszter means her zodiac sign is Pisces."

The girl raises her eyebrow, then looks us up and down before scowling. She particularly doesn't like the look of Eszter and reserves her most withering look for her.

"I am not a pagan; I am a Christian. I don't do zodiacs. They are an abomination to the Lord, and they are false idols," she scolds and turns her back on us.

Eszter is crestfallen and turns away, returning slowly to her bed.

The girl clearly hasn't finished with me, though, turning back towards me saying, "What are you doing with her?

She is a dirty junkie, and she is troublesome, making all that fuss." Her so-called Christian ethos dissipates, leaving a mean spiritedness seeping from her.

I eye her up and, trying to appeal to her better nature, say, "Can you not imagine what it must be like to be so ill, have no friend or family around you, and not understand the language? Image if it was us that had found ourselves in that situation."

She glares at me and says, "She doesn't deserve to be here." Then she turns away again.

I walk away, marvelling at how this woman can believe herself to be a "good Christian". I pass the closed curtains around Eszter's world, but as I reach my bed, she pulls them aside. Her area is by the window. It is now afternoon, and the sun streams through the glass, creating an almost biblical shaft of light that falls across her shoulders. My breath catches in my throat as I see Eszter sitting on her bed wearing a nun's wimple on her head. I have no idea where she got it, but the image is striking, and I realise that she looks uncannily like Villanelle in *Killing Eve*. Her head is bent, her hands sit palm upwards in her lap, and her lips are moving as if in prayer.

The pious young woman cannot resist a peek, and my gaze jumps between Eszter and her, wondering what will happen.

The young woman appears awestruck and says to Eszter, "Are you a nun?"

Eszter doesn't look up but nods slowly, then shoots me a sidewise look as if to say, "don't you tell". I can't hold it back any longer, and disappear behind my own curtains, stuffing the sleeve of my pj's into my mouth, hoping to stifle the laughter that is trying to escape.

The young woman spends the next two days, before her discharge, trying to ingratiate herself to Eszter with offers of chocolates and crisps. She tries to pray with Eszter, but Eszter always appears too busy talking with God to be able to do so. She continues to wear the nun's coif, clearly delighting in the attention she has found, and the extra treats go some way to satisfy her sweet tooth.

As soon as the young woman is discharged, Eszter whips off the headdress and returns to perhaps plotting her next mischievous act. Gladys and I laugh and laugh. Eszter shrugs, her wispy blonde hair framing her elfin face, and gives us a grin that for once reaches all the way to her piercing blue eyes.

A Day with the Island of Strangers

I wake with a start, still wearing my eye mask and headphones. I'd hoped music might cut out the cacophony of sounds during the night. Niela, one of the Keralite nurses, is tapping my arm. It's the early hours, and she has come to do my obs.

"Sorry to wake. Can you sit up, or your oxygen intake level will be too low?" she asks.

"Nandi (Thank you – Malayalam, Indian)," I obey, raising myself to a seating position.

Next appears Davinder, tired but smiling. She is a phlebotomist who always finds a vein but never leaves a mark. We chat. She is going home to India and is so excited to see her mum. I wish her a good trip and say, "Shukriya (Thank you – Hindi)."

Josephine arrives, as always shoes slapping the floor like wet flounder. Maria is with her, and they ask if I would like my bed made. Student nurses' chores this morning.

"Seridei (Good morning – Nigerian Izon)," I greet Josephine and then say to Maria, "Bom dia, Maria (Portuguese Brazilian)."

"Ola, uma boa noite? (Hi, did you have a good night?)" she asks.

"Mornin', mornin', ladies. Some ikkle breakfass fo u all." (Jamaican) bellows Patty, shuffling things around on her trolley and humming "Murder she wrote" by Chaka Demus.

I love this song and can't resist singing to her. "I know this little girl, her name is Maxine. Her beauty is like a bunch of roses. If I ever tell you 'bout Maxine, yuh would say I don't know what I know. Murder she wrote." She joins in the chorus.

A long shadow casts itself across my bed and I look up to see Fatima, who is the ward cleaner today. At almost seven foot tall, she is incredibly elegant in her long dark grey and black robes. She seems to hover above the lino floor, moving her broom like a Venetian gondolier as she sweeps, removing the dust grommets from under our beds.

"As-salamu alaykum, Abayo (Peace be upon you, my sister – Somali/Arabic)," I say.

She beams, flashing her glacial white teeth. It's Ramadan, and although fasting, she is still working. Tomorrow, depending on whether a new crescent moon can be seen, it could be Eid. I risk asking what food she is looking forward to, but she shakes her head, telling me that as it is just her and her sister left now, and they do not celebrate any more. I say that I am sorry and because I may not see her again before tomorrow, I wish her "Eid Mubarak (Exalted celebrations to you – Arabic)," just in case.

After breakfast, Mr Isaac the jovial porter comes, ready to take me for an ultrasound. We have met before and have had serious conversations about our mutual love of rum. He favours Guyanese, whereas I prefer Zacapa rum from Guatemala; we affably agree to disagree.

"Aw di mohnin, Mr Isaac?" I ask him (Krio – English-based Creole, Sierra Leone).

"A wel," he replies, as he pushes my wheelchair through the ward, nodding and replying to greetings and smiles from the other patients and nurses.

Mr Isaac parks my wheelchair in the ultrasound unit, hot-footing it off to another job. A young man appears, asking for my details. I take a guess that he is Filipino or maybe Malay. I go with my first instinct and say, "Kumusta Ka? (Hello, and how are you? – Tagalog- Philippines)."

I am rewarded with "Mbuti naman (I am fine)," and a toothy grin.

We chat about Palawan; I tell him how I have always wanted to snorkel there. He has been, and he says it is beautiful. Another place to visit when I am well.

As I leave, I say, "Salamat (Thank you)."

And he says, "Enjoy Palawan."

Returning to the ward, I have missed lunch. Miraculously, the nurses find a tuna mayo sandwich in fairly good condition. A clot of junior haematology doctors appears, led by Eleni the Senior Haem SpR. I hurriedly shove the sandwich into a drawer, squashing it in the process.

"Kaliméra. Ti káneis Eleni? (Good day. How are you? – Greek)" I greet her, thinking of past holidays on Greek Islands.

"Kala. Yassos, Lina (I am good. Hello, Lina)."

The junior doctors shuffle their feet, pens in clammy mitts, poised for notetaking. Eleni flicks her hand impatiently in my direction. The chosen victim places a stethoscope on my back, tapping me vigorously between the shoulder blades like a death watch beetle. While he intently listens for some non-existent infection, Eleni advises they have had luck in arranging the long-awaited biopsy on my knee, as the head radiologist agreed to stay late tonight.

This is great news; the results will determine the type of lymphoma I have. Without these, it is impossible to tailor the immunotherapy and chemo drugs which will attack the cancer with my immune system. If the biopsy were to fail, it will mean the removal of a lymph node in my neck – an unpleasant and slightly risky procedure. This area of the neck and shoulder has a mass of fragile blood vessels and nerves which could be damaged. The surgical team, my consultant and I are all not keen for this lymph node removal to take place, so it is imperative this biopsy works.

I thank Eleni profusely before she leaves. "Efcharisto poli (Thank you so much)."

Usually, after lunch there is a quietness; most patients catch forty winks and the sound of gentle snoring floats through the bay. Today is different. Feeling raw, my empathic self is unable to cope with Gladys's fears of being put in a home, not allowed to return her flat and her independence. She sits despondently in her chair, so small and shut down today. My heart aches for her.

Eszter also is unsettled. Her PICC line is infected, she is crying out in pain, and talking of suicide, saying she cannot take it anymore. As I hear Eszter, I fear what the wolf has in store for me – a world of pain. Is this how it will be once they have started my treatment? As yet it is still unclear what type of lymphoma I have. I feel impotent; the stagnancy and uncertainty grates my emotions, ramping up my anxiety. As I lay on my bed, tears track down my cheeks and pool on the pillow. I tell myself to breathe, but instead an involuntary, noisy sob escapes. The curtain is gently pulled back, and Ruth appears. Coming over, she pats my shoulder, saying, "You will be ok, we will look after you. Do not worry."

She is from Cote d'Ivoire and has a soft French accent, making her words sound like they are coated in chocolate.

"I'm sorry," I say but am unable to stop the tears and sobs.

"It's ok, let us talk. You can tell me what you are worried about."

To my surprise, she pulls up a chair, takes my hand, and looks at me directly, making sure that I understand that she is listening. She stays until I have said all I need to say and my black thoughts are lanced, leaving me calmer and ready to continue onwards, knowing this is the way it must be now, and they will start treatment when they can.

Before going, Ruth tells me to find her if I need to talk at any time. It is only when I go into the hallway and see a poster that I realise she is one of the end-of-life nurses.

As the afternoon disappears, I am taken to interventional radiology. The team is ready and waiting for me, but clearly it has been a long day. The head radiology surgeon, Sofia, explains what will happen, then makes small talk to calm my nerves. She is from Romania, has lived here for years, and likes it.

I tell her that I have been attempting to learn "hello" and "thank you" in languages of all the staff that have cared for me. Amused, she furnishes me with the Romanian words: "multumesc" (thank you) and "buna ziua" (hello). Before I go back to the ward. I thank her and her team for so kindly staying late after their busy day. The biopsy proves successful in providing the information needed.

Patty brings my pre-ordered dinner, but it's still early so I set it aside as my partner, Wendy, arrives. I recant all the "goings on" of the day, and we hope this means progress towards my treatment and escape from hospital.

As we chat, our friend Rajinder walks in. She calls out hello to other patients in the bay who recognise her from her daily visits. She has been truly amazing. Intuitively understanding that because Wendy stays for the end of visiting hours, it means she arrives home late and can be too tired to start making food herself. So, each evening, after her own working day, Rajinder pops home to collect whatever culinary delight she has made. Then she comes to the ward to drop off the meal so Wendy and I can have dinner together.

She puts down the food, saying that she will see us again tomorrow, waving away our half-hearted suggestions of her not bringing food the next day. We set up our individual meals on the bedside table like a picnic; only the gingham tablecloth is missing. I know Wendy's meal, cooked by Rajinder, will be flavoursome, delicious, and interesting – a far cry from my bland, hospital-provided offering. I may be a tad envious.

Visting hours are over, the bay is still, and the evening stretches before us.

Knock, knock, and Zeynep's head appears around the curtain.

"Nasılsın? (How are you? – Turkish),"I say.

She shakes her head slowly, her dark eyes rimmed by red. Her mother has recently passed from cancer, and she is trying to hide her grief. She says it is better to be doing something, and work is a distraction, but I know that her husband is currently jobless, so she has no option and needs to work.

I have little fist-size linen bags filled with the lavender harvest from our allotment. I sleep with them on my chest, crushing them to release the flower's aroma and help me relax. I reach into my table drawer and fish out a spare bag, offering it to Zeynep, telling her to squeeze it and then smell. She smiles, thanks me, and tucks it into her pocket. I say that I hope the night shift will be quiet.

"Yes quiet, but not too quiet." She smiles weakly.

Its 10pm, the drinks trolley has been and gone.Sweet tooth cravings of my fellow patients have been sated by the consumption of various cakes and warm milk drinks. The last obs of the night are being performed by Nadu, tonight's night shift nurse. Previously, I have mistakenly called her laddu – an Indian word meaning sweetie or dumpling. I occasionally make this error accidentally on purpose, as I know she thinks it is funny.

After finishing my obs, she brings me a little paper cup of my evening tablets and then says that if I need anything I should press the buzzer that is hanging over the top of my bed. I say "Nandi (Thank you – Malayalam – Kerala, India)," as she leaves.

This has been just one day, when just a single patient (me) has needed the attention and care of so many hospital staff.

Nurses, auxiliary staff, cleaners, doctors, porters, radiologists, phlebotomists, kitchen staff, and student nurses. These peoples of distant lands, this island of strangers that cradle us in our time of need, when our bodies – and sometimes our minds – are at their weakest. Even as my fractious self appears, they are still patient with me, showing care, respect, and making sure that I am seen and my voice heard.

We must never forget how blessed as a nation we are to have them, nor stop understanding how we and our NHS would manage without them.

Shevanti and the Television Aerial

Today I have my first chemo. It is a big day, and I need to be fitted with a dreaded cannula in one of my arms. Although the inserting of the needle is always problematic, when it's over its over, but it is the thought and feel of the damn thing in my arm which I find so intolerable!

Just before 8am, I hear the soft tread of footsteps and then see a pair of black trainers appear under the curtain around my bed. They have an 'S' on the side, and they are moving fast.

A voice says, "Knock, knock."

This is a lovely, quaint habit that many of the nurses have adopted. Of course there is no door, just a curtain, but it gives a sense of respect for the privacy of the patient, and it makes me smile every time.

Before the curtain is pulled back, I say, "Ah, sukhamano (how are you?), my favourite vampire. So, I have VIP service today, eh?"

Shevanti's head, with her Shiva-like eye makeup, appears around the edge of the curtain. As always, she has her mask on, so I cannot see her lower face, but I can see she has a twinkle in her eyes.

A few years ago, the NHS had a recruitment drive in Kerala, India, for nurses. The level of nurse training and education in Kerala is extremely high, and many of the potential nurses had excellent English, so it was remarkably successful. Hence, many Keralan nurses work throughout the UK today.

"How did you know it was me?" she laughs.

"I saw your shoes under the curtain. You have an 'S' on them for Shevanti," I say, and she laughs.

After applying EMLA cream to numb an area on my arm, she returns after a while and manages to insert the beastly cannula, hooking me up to my first six-hour chemo session. Shevanti checks in on me throughout, doing my obs: blood pressure, oxygen intake, and temperature, and always making sure I am comfortable. She pats my shoulder each time and tells me that I will be fine.

After coming back from a well-deserved afternoon break, she lets on that today is her five-year-old daughter Rani's birthday, and how she has been to the park which she loves to do. I mistakenly understand that Shevanti has seen her daughter during her break.

"No, no, she is in Kerala with my mother."

"Oh, so when was the last time you saw Rani?" I ask.

"One year ago." She produces a well-loved photo of a little girl in a silk pink dress and white shoes, standing, doll-like, on the steps of a wooden house.

"Is she like you?" I ask.

Shevanti wiggles her head back and forth in an Indian "maybe, maybe not" gesture.

"You know, powerful? Maybe she will grow up to be the prime minister of India," I tease, and we laugh.

A while later, Shevanti comes back with another bag of liquid as part of the chemo. "Raspberry juice," she says, and I nod, thinking that it doesn't look pink at all. Later, and after baffling various doctors and to the hilarity of the nurses, I realise I have the name wrong. It is, in fact, Rasburicase, which will be given to me for a few days after my chemo. This is to protect me from tumour lysis syndrome.

With chemo, tumours can break down very quickly, and in doing so, they release chemicals and cancerous cells which can affect the kidneys and cause problems with heart rhythm. From then on, whenever a nurse brings this to me, they always call it raspberry juice and chuckle. I am happy to have renamed it.

Shevanti hooks me up to the new bag, then gently takes hold of my arm with the cannula. She starts to move my arm up and down, side to side, and then in circular movements, all the while staring intently at the aerial-like contraption holding the drip bag. I suddenly get a terrible fit of the giggles.

"Shevanti, I am not a television, you know," I finally manage to say breathlessly. "Are you trying to get a good picture? What programme are looking for?"

We both crack up, laughing like lunatics until the tears of laughter are streaming down our cheeks, and I am worried that Shevanti's Shiva-like eye makeup may run.

So, thanks to her, I've survived my first chemo session, and really, it has not been too bad.

The Artful Pigeon

Since I was a child, I have been frightened of birds getting caught inside rooms. The thought of the frenetic flapping of wings and of claws caught in my hair could paralyse me with icy, clenched-teeth fear. No doubt there must have been some traumatic event that I have shelved and chosen not to remember.

During my hospital sojourn, my bed – located by the window – gave me a view over the slatey rooftops of the Victorian, brick terraced houses of Southeast London. Dawn brought the blush light of the waking sun, flooding the ward as it peeped its way past the high-rise flats overlooking the hospital like two sentinels.

The windows, which ran along the length of my bed bay, could be pushed open horizontally, and there was a little windowsill. As the weather had been warm, I considered myself to be lucky that I had the luxury of being able to push open the window for air anytime I wished, day or night.

Today I was to be hooked up once more to a drip, to protect me from the fallout of the now shrinking tumours that sat under my kneecap and groin.

"Knock, knock." Shevanti pokes her head in, her usual mask covering the lower part of her face. With her is a new student nurse.

"This is Maria, she will be shadowing me," explains Shevanti.

"Hello," says Maria, and I detect an accent.

"Shevanti is the best," I say. "She is like the professor of nurses. Where are you from, Maria? I can tell that you have a little accent."

"I am from Sao Paulo, Brazil," she says.

"Ah, bom dia (good morning), Maria," I reply. Shevanti gives me a look to say "you are showing off again". But I don't care.

"Voce fala portugues? (Do you speak Portuguese?)" asks Maria.

"No, just a few words. But you can teach me more."

They work together to change my bed. The lymphoma makes me sweat profusely in the early hours, and at times my bed is drenched as if a bucket of water has been thrown over it. Each morning, and if necessary, sometimes at night, the nurses dutifully and without hesitation change the sheets and refresh my bed.

Shevanti and Maria attach the new drip bag to the existing cannula in my arm. It will take about an hour to drip through. They ask me if there is anything I need and if I want the open window closed a little. I tell them to please leave it open, as it's warm and I am enjoying the breeze. They make sure I have a full beaker of water and a well plenished jug on my table on the side of my "good", non-cannulated arm, then leave.

I decide to take a doze. It's worth taking any opportunity to catch up with the often-missed sleep from the sometimes noisy, busy nights. But it seems no time at all before I hear a scratching and then a cooing noise. My eyes fly open to be accosted by the sight of a pigeon sitting on the windowsill, both its head and body inside.

I scream, but the pigeon is a battle-hardened individual and continues to coo then makes to come in further. Without hesitation, I pick up the plastic beaker of water and hurl it at the would-be interloper. Miraculously, I hit it on the head, knocking it out. I hear the pad, pad of running feet encased in trainers, as both Shevanti and Maria burst through the curtains. No mention of "knock, knock" this time. I realise that I am still screaming.

"Are you ok?" they say in unison. Both instinctively look at the drip but see that it is fine and still running through. "What's happened?"

"That!" I say, pointing to the window.

Shevanti, followed by Maria, goes to the window to see the stunned, prone pigeon lying on the windowsill. As they watch, it shakes and uprights itself, regains its composure, and flies off.

They take in the plastic beaker lying empty on the floor beneath the window. Bemused, they ask, "What did you do?"

"I threw the water beaker at it! I hate pigeons, and it was trying to get in!"

"OMG, you tried to kill a pigeon!" They both think this is hilarious.

"They come in here all the time; we are always having to chase them," says Shevanti, really laughing, tears streaming down her now soggy mask.

"Coo, coo," she says and flaps her arms.

"Don't!" I say. "It's not funny." But I can't convince them otherwise, and they go off making cooing noises and laughing. Before they leave, they give me a fresh beaker of water.

"In case another pigeon comes, and it is thirsty," they say.

From now on, I insist that the window is only open the width of a pigeon's head. But each time Shevanti or Maria enter my curtained enclave, they say "coo, coo" instead of "knock, knock".

Queen Rat and Lemon Drizzle Cake

Eszter has been coveting a bracelet, strung with elastic, and bejewelled with small plastic, orange flowers. She tells me that it reminds her of the trance music and dancing at the full-moon parties when she was in Thailand.

"I vant it, will make me happys," she tells me, as we chat one morning before breakfast. There is a woman, a fellow patient, in another bay area of the ward, that she has talked to a couple of times who has it on her wrist.

"Will she give it to you?" I ask.

Eszter tuts and looks at me like I am a total innocent.

"No, she vill swap!" she hisses in a slightly irritated tone.

I am worried. I know that Eszter has a problem with drugs and booze. Sometimes, to take a break from the ward's stifling micro world, she disappears downstairs. There are nesting geese on a shed roof that overlooks the water meadow running behind the hospital. Eszter has taken photos to show me and has been delighted in my interest. Sadly, though, she is often targeted by pushers on these escapes.

On a couple of occasions, she has returned a "little bit out of it". This initially makes her happy but then ultimately sad. I have grown fond of her and it's difficult to see her spending days admonishing herself when this happens.

"What does she want to swap it for?" I ask Eszter.

She looks around furtively to see if anyone is in earshot, and then in hushed tones says, "Lemon cake."

"How much lemon cake?" I ask.

"Six pieces," she says mournfully.

If you have been an inpatient for any length of time in this hospital, you know that at 7pm each evening the trolley is pushed through the ward and bedtime hot drinks are doled out. Gladys always has "ot shocolate" and Eszter the same, but insists three spoons of sugar are added, despite it being overly sweet already. It must make her teeth itch. Not understanding the need for such saccharine sweet morsels before bedtime, I always decline.

In addition to the hot drinks, there is always cake on offer: chocolate, fruitcake, and the ever-popular lemon drizzle cake. The lemon cake has reached some dizzy height of mystical longing, with most of the patients fanatically believing that it is far superior to anything else they might be given. The problem is that, as we are the last bay on the ward, often this much lorded cake has run out.

Each evening Eszter trills, "Lemon cake, please."

Eight out of ten times she is met with, "No lemon cake; all gone. You want chocolate or fruit cake?"

"No," she replies. "Nothing."

So, with this in mind, I wonder how we are going to purloin six pieces of this valuable cake so she can procure her "happy bracelet". Eszter knows I do not eat cake – not even the supposedly heavenly lemon drizzle cake. I sense she has a plan. Like Queen Rat, she would survive in any environment.

"I shink you ask for de lemon cake. Sey like you, sey will give you," she says sagely.

That evening, we test out the plan, but of course it fails. As predicted, lemon cake has all been taken by the other patients served before us. Eszter is sulking and looks miserable. Marsha, the evening trolley lady, takes pity on her, kindly saying that she will save some lemon cake for her tomorrow.

Eszter claps her hands like a child. "Yes, yes, two pieces please."

The evening groans on as usual then quietens down as we prepare for slumber. Around 2am there is a commotion, and a bed with a moaning patient is sardined into the bay. The new patient is clearly in a lot of pain, crying out as the nurses try to fit cannulas to get soothing drugs into her as quickly as possible. This level of discomfort usually means a sickle cell patient in crisis. This happens when blood vessels to a part of the body become blocked by the unusually sickle-shaped red blood cells. The pain is very severe and can last hours, days, or weeks. We lie wincing in our beds and wishing for it to pass quickly for her. Eventually, the nurses win, the drugs kick in, her gasps of pain subside, and finally we all sleep.

The next morning, we hear our new companion before we see her. She is in a much better state than she was last night. Her voice would have benefitted a career on the stage and seems to have no low volume switch.

I am just at the bottom of Gladys's bed, saying my morning greetings to her, when she tuts and says in her usual stage whisper, "She's got a voice like Gracie."

I take a guess that she's probably referring to Gracie Fields and her "cracked voice" when she was singing her song "Sally".

A nurse walks into the bay and goes towards the new patient's bed.

"Chantal, how are you doing this morning? Oh my, why do you have all these phones? What are you doing? You need to rest. Come now, put them away."

"No, I need to have them. I'm an influencer, it's my job," says Chantal.

Gladys beckons me closer. "Er, what she says? Did she say she'd got the influenza? She better not come near me wiv dat!"

"No, she said she's an influencer," I try to explain in hushed tones.

"What?" Gladys barks.

"She gives her opinion on things like fashions, food, and stuff. People follow what she says, so she influences what they buy, wear, and eat," I say trying, to be helpful.

Gladys sniffs and says, "Why they listen to 'er then? Flibbertigibbet!"

"I don't know, Gladys." I move on, hearing the breakfast trolley in the distance.

As the trolley appears, Chantal is still talking loudly, switching between various social media accounts on her phone. Occasionally she says, "No, I don't want them to know all my stuff!"

This seems incongruous, given her chosen career. As soon as she realises that breakfast is imminent, she shuts down her conversations and calls out, "Hey, hey, whatcha have? I am sooooo hungry."

Patty, our breakfast lady, is already standing beside Gladys's bed, just about to take her breakfast order.

"S'or rite," says Gladys. "Do 'er first, poor cow, she 'ad a bad night."

Patty moves towards Chantal. "Wha' you like for breakfass?" she asks, the Jamaican lilt coming through.

"I want four white toasts, some porridge with hot milk, and tea with milk and two sugar," says Chantal, who is clearly ravenous after her ordeal of the previous night.

"You gonna eats all dat?" says Patty

"Yep, I am sooooo hungry. Also, you got any snacks? You know, for the day?" asks Chantal.

Patty bends and opens the "secret" doors under the trolley. "Let me see, I have biscuits and some cake."

I hear a sharp intake of breath from Eszter's direction.

"What cake you have?" Asks Chantal.

"I have fruitcake and chocolate." There is a sigh from Eszter. "Oh, and lemon cake," says Patty.

I expect to see Eszter throwing herself off her bed in Patty's direction, but somehow, she holds back, and we hear Chantal say, "I'll have chocolate."

I swear I hear Eszter jumping up and down in relief.

After Patty has given Chantal her gargantuan breakfast and snacks, she moves over to Gladys and then comes to my curtains. "Morning," she says.

"Hello Patty, morning. How are you on this lovely day?" I say, determined to lull her into good spirts.

"All good." She smiles and takes my breakfast order of brown toast and black tea. As she puts the plate and mug on my bedside table, I venture, "Umm, would you happen to have any of that lemon cake spare? I have heard it's good, but I've never tried it."

"Let me see," she says with a conspiratorial wink.

She returns with three pieces of cigarette packet-sized lemon cake. "Here. I knows it always run out, so you never get' any. T'will keep a coople o' days."

"Oh Patty, you are a star. Thank you so much," I say, flashing my best smile.

She moves on to Eszter. "Yes, I have some for you, too, don't you worry."

"Oh, my Gott, tank you so much," says Eszter.

As soon as Patty leaves, Eszter and I meet to count the loot, but between us we have five pieces instead of the required six.

"Maybe she will take five pieces for the bracelet?" I say hopefully.

Eszter shakes her head. "No, must be six."

I have a brainwave. I take my crutches and hobble over to Gladys. "Hey, Gladys, did you get any lemon cake just now?"

"Yeah, but I likes fruitcake. She just put it on me table and went before I could tell 'er."

"Tell you what, can I have it and I'll get you an extra piece of fruitcake to go with your hot chocolate tonight?" I try hopefully.

"Al-rite, go on then."

I take the lemon cake before she can change her mind, and go back to Eszter, holding out my hand to show her what I have. As I hand over all the cake, Eszter takes the hoard and disappears out of the bay, onto the ward, lickety-split, like a jet-propelled elf. Five minutes later she is back, beaming. I hear a click-click and see the orange plastic flowers of her treasure. She has a Cheshire cat smile across her face; small wins can be sweet. She flicks the bracelet adorning her painfully slim wrist, dangling and swinging her feet back and forth like a child as she sits on her bed, her small orbit somehow a little richer today.

Josephine's Treat

My partner is sitting by my bed. Today I am due to go home, and we are waiting for my "meds" to be delivered from the pharmacy. I am not convinced it is going to happen and have not changed yet into my "outside wear".

I have been an inpatient for three-and-a-half weeks, and I fear that I may have become institutionalised. I wonder if I might soon be wearing a little woollen hat, rocking back and forth, humming "Jerusalem" to myself. I find it disturbing that I have now completely handed over my general wellbeing. Even more potently alarming, I recognise the squeak of the wonky wheel on the food trolley when it is being pushed down the ward, wake automatically at 6am, and find myself waiting for the "prickers", who will not visit me this morning.

Although I so want to get home and sit in the garden where my partner has planted my favourite flowers, there is part of me that is shocked in the understanding that I will miss the daily rhythms, the staff who have been so caring of me, and my fellow patients.

During my stay there have been three student nurses from Nigeria and Brazil. They are all in their final year, and the potential they show to be wonderful caring nurses of tomorrow is clear. Today Josephine is working, busy and helpful, with shoes rather than trainers, which make a reassuring slapping noise as she walks. She is the most gregarious of the three, with a smile that is huge and seems to fill the room. From the Niger Delta, she is Ijaw – one of the oldest ethnic groups – and is the only Nigerian nurse here who speaks the dialect, Izon. I have failed miserably to remember the few greetings she has taught me, but she has kindly accepted Yoruba greetings without not too much tutting and tongue clicking. We have had so many chats about Niger Delta food. I have heard mouthwatering descriptions of banga soup and ofada stew until I had to beg her to stop when the chemo made me feel so queasy.

All the nurses know how much I hate the cannula that is currently sitting in my vein like some alien, metallic creature. They have decided to give Josephine the "treat" of removing it before I leave.

The curtains are abruptly yanked back, and there is that wonderful smile. Josephine says, "E karro (Good morning to you)."

I decide to risk an answer. "Bawo ni? (How are you?)"

"Mo wa daada (I am good)."

She has decided this is enough showing off and lapses into English. She beams her pulchritudinous smile and says in a booming voice that is almost biblical, "E, today I have come to make you free and take away your pain!"

"Oh God, what are you going to do to me now?" I say in mock alarm.

She laughs joyously. "I will be the one to take away the cannula."

"Whaa! Now I know that your fellow nurses are spoiling me on my last day by sending me you. This is VIP treatment," I say to her delight.

"One moment," she says and steps outside the curtains again.

Quickly, I grab my phone and hurriedly tap onto my music, finding the song I want, and then hide it in my cannula free hand. Josephine returns, struggling into her blue non-latex gloves, pulls the curtain around again, and then picks up my hand. She slowly draws out the demon cannula and says triumphantly, "There, you are free!"

I hit the music button, and Eddy Kenzo's Afro beats song "Blessings" fills the ward. Josephine squeals and starts to dance, with my partner joining in, and me fanny dancing in the bed, all of us laughing and whooping. We hear quick footsteps, and the curtain is pulled back to reveal some of the other nurses who smile, clap their hands, and for a few moments join in the dancing. I can see that the other patients are joining in too, nodding to the music before I respectfully turn it off and some normality returns.

Shevanti is standing in the doorway watching. She shakes her head, and then just before she moves away, she pulls down her mask as she is turning, and I can see that she too is smiling.

Josephine, still grinning, says to me, "You know Eddy Kenzo is Ugandan, not Nigerian."

I look at her and say, "Well, you are not putting the cannula back in, so you can take it out again with Nigerian dance music playing!"

She laughs and walks away with her flipper-like shoes slapping the floor. And yes, I do feel liberated and ready to go home.

Aftermath

Today I sit in our garden, filled with favourite flowers planted by my partner, hearing birds twittering and seeing the sudden flash of green, as thuggish parakeets colour the grey sky. The moggies have punished me for my absence but finally relented, possibly due to the extra treats I gave them.

I have just completed my fourth chemo/immunotherapy session and two PET scans, which show my response to treatment has been extremely good; the tumours have shrunk and are now inactive. This has happened far quicker than anticipated and beyond our expectations, but we know that it is still a long road.

The side-effects of the treatment are gruelling and relentless, but they follow a recognised pattern, so are not so alarming anymore. After chemo I am exhausted, having been pumped full of powerful and toxic tumour-killing drugs, but I am given four days of steroids so cannot sleep. Imbued with faux energy, I find myself book writing, whittling wood, and jam making – keeping myself busy. Then, crashing hard, I sink quickly into a nadir that lasts several days, my appetite dies, and I feel nauseous. I am dragged into a fathomless hole, a black negativity that leaves me weeping constantly and in absentia.

Unfortunately, this coincides with the neutropenia shots. I must inject myself with these for a seemingly endless eight days, starting from the fifth day after chem. These aid my bone marrow in boosting the production of white blood cells to fight infection. But I find these days hard on my already chemical-laden body, with pains in the bones of my chest, ribs, and back that resemble brain freeze after gulping an ice-cold drink.

The first time this happened; I thought I was having a heart attack but now know this means that it will pass in two or three days. Then suddenly, like a phoenix, I arise, myself again until the next session and a repeat of the pattern.

An interesting side-effect has been the change in colour of my eyes. I am brown eyed normally but was alarmed to see that in hospital, after the first chemo session, they changed to a deep ocean blue for a few days. On my second session, they went "Bowie" – one pupil was dark blue and the other brown, which I quite liked and felt gave me some kudos. Recently, and a little disappointingly, they were just slightly greener. A friend told me this can be an effect of immunotherapy but will not last, so it seems that I will not retain this potentially unique superpower.

Less hirsute than I was, my eyebrows are lost, my eyelashes are virtually gone, and I am totally bald – a slap head. I accept compliments that I "rock" the look, having a nice-shaped head. Recently a black vest, Sigourney Weaver-like, has become my fashionista style, although her *Aliens'* Ellen Ripley character is far fiercer than I could ever be. Amusingly, I am slightly preoccupied by the idea that a passing stranger my stick their fingers in my ears and treat me like a bowling ball. My hair will grow back but might be wiry and possibly not the same colour. Most definitely not the Sofia Loren locks I always dreamed of.

And what of Gladys and Eszter? Sadly, I have no further news of them since I left the ward. I hope they are doing well, Gladys in her freshly refurbished flat and Eszter somewhere that is safe for her. They will always be with me, and I will never be able to see a nun or hear the word "exactly" without thinking of them.

So, things are toddling along nicely, and I no longer believe that I am going to die imminently. Taking stock, I appreciate my good, rich life, full of possibilities and potential. I recognise just how fortunate I am to have my partner, family, and friends, who surround me and hold me in a supportive mantle. During this darkest of times, they have shown me how loved and cared for I am, pushing me through to positivity and hopefulness. After all, where would any of us be without hope and love?

Acknowledgments and Thanks

I would like firstly and foremostly to thank my partner, Wendy, who has shown me such love, caring, and strength during this awful time. There have been days when it has all seemed too big to cope with, but she has reminded me of all the plans and the things we have yet to do, pulling me onward towards them.

My mother, sister, and nieces have also been there for us, taking on the task of passing information of my progress to family near and far, and relaying back to me good wishes, thoughts, and blessing from all over the world.

I would also like to thank my friends, some who have reconnected from the past. They have steadfastly been so supportive and caring, sending me caring messages, cards, and healing gifts for my heart, body, and soul. I have received much needed words of encouragement and love as I disappear into the black hole of the chemo nadir and then rejoicing as I reappear.

Special thanks go to Angela, who listened with patience to my ideas of how the wolf should appear and then produced the perfect likeness for the front of my book.

I would also like to acknowledge with appreciation Michael Rosen for writing the poem "Island of Strangers" about his time in hospital. It resonated with me so strongly, capturing what I try to express in my book about my care and staff that work in the NHS, but also sadly the xenophobia that is still prevalent in our sometimes so ungrateful society.

Appreciation to Melanie and the team at Grosvenor House Publishing for their patience and guidance.

Abounding gratitude to Dr Tullie Yeghen, Dr Chandima and the dedicated team of Haematologists at Lewisham Hospital without whom, I feel, I would not be here.

Lastly, I cannot express my gratitude enough to the wonderful staff of Lewisham Hospital. The dedication, care, warmth, and respect they showed far surpassed my expectations. I have heard others say being an inpatient elsewhere was harrowing, that they were treated like "a piece of meat", unheard and unseen, but this was never the case for me at Lewisham Hospital. Meeting the staff and patients that I did was an enriching and life-affirming experience for me.

About the Author

Lina Lazaretto is the nom de plume of Corinna Percario. I was born in Kuala Lumpur, to an unusually calm but charismatic Italian father and the "force of nature" which is my English Mother. I live in London with my long-suffering partner and three feisty, dictatorial felines. Fortunate to have travelled all over the world, I have lived in palaces, country estates, and squats. When there was such a thing, I worked for the East German tourist office in London, then in the travel industry for a few decades before working in the NHS – ironically, in Oncology and Haematology – before finally escaping. Rushing into retirement early, hell for leather, happily trying to catch a few golden years before my decrepitude.

My parents – my father a chef and mother a general "fixer" – worked for the British High commission in both Nigeria and Malaysia in the 60s. Each country, excited by their imminent independence and the new possibilities coming their way, held the fondest memories for my parents. As a child, I danced to the Nigerian Highlife music and thought the Beatles were glamorous Chinese women with beehive hairdos, silk dresses, and stiletto shoes. Later, when older, I realised that my father disliked the Beatles intensely and instead preferred the Beatles tribute band called The Korean Kittens.

While my parents worked in Kuala Lumpur, I was left in the care of Mai Lei, my ama; hence my first language was

Hainan Chinese. As well as teaching me to speak, I am forever indebted to her for showing me how to wield chopsticks at under two years old, way before mastering cumbersome knives and folks. It proved to be a boon for business trips into China when I was working in travel.

My parents found it difficult to communicate with me, and there exists grainy cinefilm of me standing on a chair in a downtown KL restaurant, chinwagging with the waiters in Chinese. They were amused but ultimately patient with this blonde, Shirley Temple-like infant chatting away to them.

When we returned to a country estate in rural Wiltshire, I was distressed at aged four to come across the loud, ruddy, grubby farm children and realise I was not Chinese. It took a lot for my mother to placate and convince me otherwise. Years later, managing an amazing team of staff from all over Southeast Asian and China, they decided to make me "honorary" Chinese, and I was extremely touched to be bestowed with such an extraordinary gift.

Afterwards, living and attending school in Switzerland, having Italian family and friends from all over the world, I picked up a few handy European languages. These have always aided me to smooth the paths of conversations in my travels and explorations. I feel it is always respectful to be able to at least thank and greet someone in their own language.

I guess then, with this background, it is not surprising that I love the cultural fruit salad of London, feeling at home sitting on a bus travelling through Southeast London and absorbing the many tongues of the folks around me. The melodies and undulations of each language delight me, making me wonder if the conversations are intense discussion about the universe or just what might be for dinner. This is what makes me feel happy, vibrant, and enriched.

I believe with all my heart that I am so very blessed to call this my home, and to have the chance to meet and learn from the people that surround me every day. I love each possibility of hearing someone's story, and learning of their culture, homeland, and life. How lucky I am.